VEGAN COOKBOOK

HEALTHY PLANT-BASED RECIPES WITH EASY INSTRUCTIONS

SARAH NEVINS

Table of Contents

Introduction

Veganism is a type of diet that can be adapted for any age and gender. Research has shown that going on a vegan diet can help lower cholesterol levels. It also helps the dieter avoid certain types of diseases such as type 2 diabetes, heart disease, hypertension and certain types of cancer.

As always, you'll want to start out gradually by taking it step by step. Most diets fail when the person tries to do too much and expect too much too soon. The best way to get on the diet is to take baby steps to help the dieter adapt to this new lifestyle in the long run. Some of these steps include removing meat and any animal products one meal at a time. You can also avoid meat for certain meals of the day.

Another step that you can take in your journey towards having a vegan lifestyle is to hang out with like minded people. Spend time with vegans in forums and especially in groups. This helps you learn and adapt best practices as well as share your thoughts and opinions with other vegans.

Many people believe that vegans lack variety in their diet due to the absence of meat and dairy products. Nothing could be further from the truth. Having a vegan diet actually allows the person to experience a wider variety of food as he starts to try a wide array of fruits, vegetables, grains, seeds and pulses. These types of food are filled with micronutrients and fiber that are not present in meat and dairy products.

Many have also been led to believe that a vegan diet lacks certain macronutrients and minerals such as protein and calcium however there's a wider array of vegetables and beans that could easily replace meat and dairy products. Tofu for instance is rich in protein.

Grilled Edamame Beans and Zucchini

Ingredients

20 pcs. Edamame Beans

1 lb zucchini, sliced lengthwise into shorter sticks

1 lb green bell peppers, sliced into wide strips

1 large red onion, cut into 1/2 inch thick rounds

1/3 cup Italian parsley or basil, finely chopped

Dressing Ingredients:

6 tbsp. extra virgin olive oil

1 tsp. onion powder

Sea salt, to taste

3 tbsp. distilled white vinegar

1 tsp. Dijon mustard

Combine all of the dressing ingredients thoroughly.

Preheat your grill to low heat and grease the grates.

Layer the vegetables grill for 12 minutes per side, until tender flipping once.

Brush with the marinade/ dressing ingredients

Grilled Cabbage and Bell Peppers

Ingredients

1 medium Cabbage sliced

1 lb green bell peppers, sliced into wide strips

1 large red onion, cut into 1/2 inch thick rounds

1/3 cup Italian parsley or basil, finely chopped

Dressing Ingredients

6 tbsp. olive oil

1 tsp. garlic powder

1 tsp. onion powder

Sea salt, to taste

3 tbsp. white wine vinegar

1 tsp. English mustard

Combine all of the dressing ingredients thoroughly.

Preheat your grill to low heat and grease the grates.

Layer the vegetables grill for 12 minutes per side, until tender flipping once.

Brush with the marinade/ dressing ingredients

Grilled Okra and Zucchini

Ingredients

10 pcs. Okra

1 lb zucchini, sliced lengthwise into shorter sticks

10 pcs. Brussel Sprouts

1 large red onion, cut into 1/2 inch thick rounds

1/3 cup Italian parsley or basil, finely chopped

Dressing Ingredients

6 tbsp. olive oil

3 dashes of Tabasco hot sauce

Sea salt, to taste

3 tbsp. white wine vinegar

1 tsp. Egg-free mayonnaise

Combine all of the dressing ingredients thoroughly.

Preheat your grill to low heat and grease the grates.

Layer the vegetables grill for 12 minutes per side, until tender flipping once.

Brush with the marinade/ dressing ingredients

Grilled Artichoke and Romaine Lettuce

Ingredients

1 pc. Artichoke

1 bunch of Romaine Lettuce leaves

2 medium Carrots, cut lengthwise and cut in half

4 large Tomatoes, sliced thick

Dressing Ingredients

6 tbsp. extra virgin olive oil

Sea salt, to taste

3 tbsp. Balsamic vinegar

1 tsp. Dijon mustard

Combine all of the dressing ingredients thoroughly.

Preheat your grill to low heat and grease the grates.

Layer the vegetables grill for 12 minutes per side, until tender flipping once.

Brush with the marinade/ dressing ingredients

Grilled Kale and Bell Peppers

Ingredients

1 bunch of Kale

1 lb green bell peppers, sliced into wide strips

1 large red onion, cut into 1/2 inch thick rounds

1/3 cup Italian parsley or basil, finely chopped

Dressing Ingredients

6 tbsp. extra virgin olive oil

Sea salt, to taste

1 tsp. onion powder

1/2 tsp. Herbs de Provence

3 tbsp. white vinegar

1 tsp. Dijon mustard

Combine all of the dressing ingredients thoroughly.

Preheat your grill to low heat and grease the grates.

Layer the vegetables grill for 12 minutes per side, until tender flipping once.

Brush with the marinade/ dressing ingredients

Grilled Beets and Broccolini Florets

Ingredients

5 pcs. Beets

1 lb green bell peppers, sliced into wide strips

10 Broccolini Florets

10 pcs. Brussel Sprouts

1 large red onion, cut into 1/2 inch thick rounds

1/3 cup Italian parsley or basil, finely chopped

Dressing Ingredients

6 tbsp. extra virgin olive oil

Sea salt, to taste

3 tbsp. apple cider vinegar

1 tbsp. honey

1 tsp. Egg-free mayonnaise

Combine all of the dressing ingredients thoroughly.

Preheat your grill to low heat and grease the grates.

Layer the vegetables grill for 12 minutes per side, until tender flipping once.

Brush with the marinade/ dressing ingredients

Grilled Edamame Beans and Romaine Lettuce

Ingredients

20 pcs. Edamame Beans

1 bunch of Romaine Lettuce leaves

2 medium Carrots, cut lengthwise and cut in half

4 large Tomatoes, sliced thick

Dressing Ingredients:

6 tbsp. extra virgin olive oil

1 tsp. onion powder

Sea salt, to taste

3 tbsp. distilled white vinegar

1 tsp. Dijon mustard

Combine all of the dressing ingredients thoroughly.

Preheat your grill to low heat and grease the grates.

Layer the vegetables grill for 12 minutes per side, until tender flipping once.

Brush with the marinade/ dressing ingredients

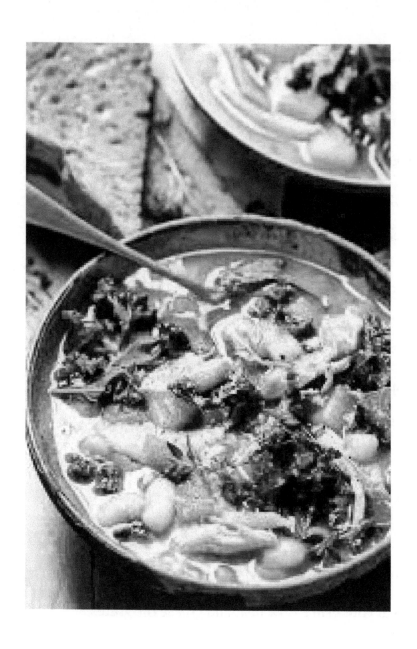

Grilled Cabbage and Green Bell Peppers

Ingredients

1 medium Cabbage sliced

1 lb green bell peppers, sliced into wide strips

1 large red onion, cut into 1/2 inch thick rounds

1/3 cup Italian parsley or basil, finely chopped

Dressing Ingredients

6 tbsp. extra virgin olive oil

Sea salt, to taste

3 tbsp. Balsamic vinegar

1 tsp. Dijon mustard

Combine all of the dressing ingredients thoroughly.

Preheat your grill to low heat and grease the grates.

Layer the vegetables grill for 12 minutes per side, until tender flipping once.

Brush with the marinade/ dressing ingredients

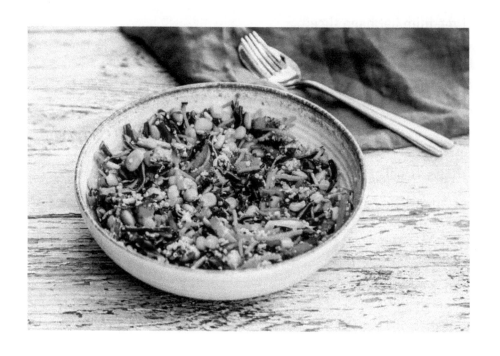

Grilled Zucchini and Cabbage

Ingredients

1 lb zucchini, sliced lengthwise into shorter sticks

1 medium Cabbage sliced

1 large red onion, cut into 1/2 inch thick rounds

1/3 cup Italian parsley or basil, finely chopped

10 Broccolini Florets

10 pcs. Brussel Sprouts

Dressing Ingredients

6 tbsp. olive oil

3 dashes of Tabasco hot sauce

Sea salt, to taste

3 tbsp. white wine vinegar

1 tsp. Egg-free mayonnaise

Combine all of the dressing ingredients thoroughly.

Preheat your grill to low heat and grease the grates.

Layer the vegetables grill for 12 minutes per side, until tender flipping once.

Brush with the marinade/ dressing ingredients

Grilled Okra and Red Onions

Ingredients

10 pcs. Okra

1 large red onion, cut into 1/2 inch thick rounds

1/3 cup Italian parsley or basil, finely chopped

Dressing Ingredients

6 tbsp. olive oil

1 tsp. garlic powder

1 tsp. onion powder

Sea salt, to taste

3 tbsp. white wine vinegar

1 tsp. English mustard

Combine all of the dressing ingredients thoroughly.

Preheat your grill to low heat and grease the grates.

Layer the vegetables grill for 12 minutes per side, until tender flipping once.

Brush with the marinade/ dressing ingredients

Grilled Artichokes and Red Onion

Ingredients

1 pc. Artichoke

1 large red onion, cut into 1/2 inch thick rounds

1/3 cup Italian parsley or basil, finely chopped

Dressing Ingredients

6 tbsp. extra virgin olive oil

Sea salt, to taste

3 tbsp. apple cider vinegar

1 tbsp. honey

1 tsp. Egg-free mayonnaise

Combine all of the dressing ingredients thoroughly.

Preheat your grill to low heat and grease the grates.

Layer the vegetables grill for 12 minutes per side, until tender flipping once.

Brush with the marinade/ dressing ingredients

28

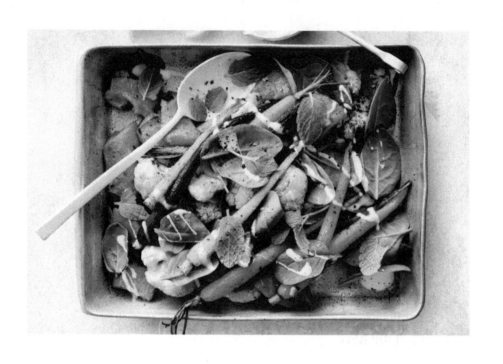

Grilled Kale and Romaine Lettuce

Ingredients

1 bunch of Kale

1 bunch of Romaine Lettuce leaves

2 medium Carrots, cut lengthwise and cut in half

4 large Tomatoes, sliced thick

1/3 cup Italian parsley or basil, finely chopped

Dressing Ingredients

6 tbsp. extra virgin olive oil

Sea salt, to taste

3 tbsp. Balsamic vinegar

1 tsp. Dijon mustard

Combine all of the dressing ingredients thoroughly.

Preheat your grill to low heat and grease the grates.

Layer the vegetables grill for 12 minutes per side, until tender flipping once.

Brush with the marinade/ dressing ingredients

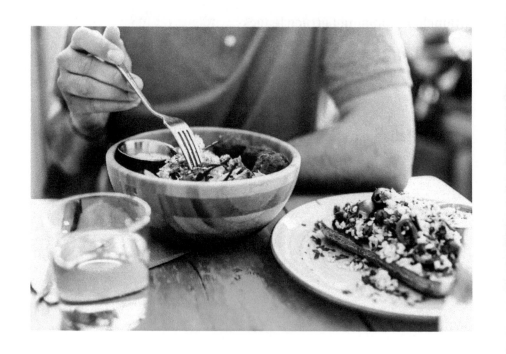

Grilled Beets and Carrots

Ingredients

5 pcs. Beets

1 bunch of Romaine Lettuce leaves

2 medium Carrots, cut lengthwise and cut in half

4 large Tomatoes, sliced thick

1/3 cup Italian parsley or basil, finely chopped

Dressing Ingredients:

6 tbsp. extra virgin olive oil

1 tsp. onion powder

Sea salt, to taste

3 tbsp. distilled white vinegar

1 tsp. Dijon mustard

Combine all of the dressing ingredients thoroughly.

Preheat your grill to low heat and grease the grates.

Layer the vegetables grill for 12 minutes per side, until tender flipping once.

Brush with the marinade/ dressing ingredients

Grilled Baby Carrots and Onion

Ingredients

8 pcs. baby carrots

1 large red onion, cut into 1/2 inch thick rounds

1/3 cup Italian parsley or basil, finely chopped

Dressing Ingredients

6 tbsp. extra virgin olive oil

Sea salt, to taste

1 tsp. onion powder

1/2 tsp. Herbs de Provence

3 tbsp. white vinegar

1 tsp. Dijon mustard

Combine all of the dressing ingredients thoroughly.

Preheat your grill to low heat and grease the grates.

Layer the vegetables grill for 12 minutes per side, until tender flipping once.

Brush with the marinade/ dressing ingredients

Grilled Baby Corn and Broccolini Florets

Ingredients

10 pcs. baby corn

10 Broccolini Florets

10 pcs. Brussel Sprouts

1 large red onion, cut into 1/2 inch thick rounds

1/3 cup Italian parsley or basil, finely chopped

Dressing Ingredients

6 tbsp. olive oil

3 dashes of Tabasco hot sauce

Sea salt, to taste

3 tbsp. white wine vinegar

1 tsp. Egg-free mayonnaise

Combine all of the dressing ingredients thoroughly.

Preheat your grill to low heat and grease the grates.

Layer the vegetables grill for 12 minutes per side, until tender flipping once.

Brush with the marinade/ dressing ingredients

Grilled Artichoke Hearts

Ingredients

1 cup artichoke hearts

1 bunch of Romaine Lettuce leaves

2 medium Carrots, cut lengthwise and cut in half

4 large Tomatoes, sliced thick

1 large red onion, cut into 1/2 inch thick rounds

1/3 cup Italian parsley or basil, finely chopped

Dressing Ingredients

6 tbsp. olive oil

1 tsp. garlic powder

1 tsp. onion powder

Sea salt, to taste

3 tbsp. white wine vinegar

1 tsp. English mustard

Combine all of the dressing ingredients thoroughly.

Preheat your grill to low heat and grease the grates.

Layer the vegetables grill for 12 minutes per side, until tender flipping once.

Brush with the marinade/ dressing ingredients

Grilled Beets and Asparagus

Ingredients

5 pcs. Beets

10 pcs. Asparagus

1 bunch of Romaine Lettuce leaves

2 medium Carrots, cut lengthwise and cut in half

4 large Tomatoes, sliced thick

1 lb green bell peppers, sliced into wide strips

1 large red onion, cut into 1/2 inch thick rounds

1/3 cup Italian parsley or basil, finely chopped

Dressing Ingredients

6 tbsp. extra virgin olive oil

Sea salt, to taste

3 tbsp. apple cider vinegar

1 tbsp. honey

1 tsp. Egg-free mayonnaise

Combine all of the dressing ingredients thoroughly.

Preheat your grill to low heat and grease the grates.

Layer the vegetables grill for 12 minutes per side, until tender flipping once.

Brush with the marinade/ dressing ingredients

Grilled Kale

Ingredients

1 bunch of Kale

1/3 cup Italian parsley or basil, finely chopped

Dressing Ingredients

6 tbsp. extra virgin olive oil

Sea salt, to taste

3 tbsp. Balsamic vinegar

1 tsp. Dijon mustard

Combine all of the dressing ingredients thoroughly.

Preheat your grill to low heat and grease the grates.

Layer the vegetables grill for 12 minutes per side, until tender flipping once.

Brush with the marinade/ dressing ingredients

Grilled Artichoke

Ingredients

1 pc. Artichoke

1/3 cup Italian parsley or basil, finely chopped

Dressing Ingredients:

6 tbsp. extra virgin olive oil

1 tsp. onion powder

Sea salt, to taste

3 tbsp. distilled white vinegar

1 tsp. Dijon mustard

Combine all of the dressing ingredients thoroughly.

Preheat your grill to low heat and grease the grates.

Layer the vegetables grill for 12 minutes per side, until tender flipping once.

Brush with the marinade/ dressing ingredients

Grilled Okra and Asparagus

Ingredients

10 pcs. Okra

10 pcs. Asparagus

1 bunch of Romaine Lettuce leaves

2 medium Carrots, cut lengthwise and cut in half

4 large Tomatoes, sliced thick

Dressing Ingredients

6 tbsp. olive oil

1 tsp. garlic powder

1 tsp. onion powder

Sea salt, to taste

3 tbsp. white wine vinegar

1 tsp. English mustard

Combine all of the dressing ingredients thoroughly.

Preheat your grill to low heat and grease the grates.

Layer the vegetables grill for 12 minutes per side, until tender flipping once.

Brush with the marinade/ dressing ingredients

Grilled Cabbage and Romaine Lettuce

Ingredients

1 medium Cabbage sliced

1 bunch of Romaine Lettuce leaves

2 medium Carrots, cut lengthwise and cut in half

4 large Tomatoes, sliced thick

1 large red onion, cut into 1/2 inch thick rounds

1/3 cup Italian parsley or basil, finely chopped

Dressing Ingredients

6 tbsp. olive oil

3 dashes of Tabasco hot sauce

Sea salt, to taste

3 tbsp. white wine vinegar

1 tsp. Egg-free mayonnaise

Combine all of the dressing ingredients thoroughly.

Preheat your grill to low heat and grease the grates.

Layer the vegetables grill for 12 minutes per side, until tender flipping once.

Brush with the marinade/ dressing ingredients

Grilled Edamame Beans and Bell Peppers

Ingredients

20 pcs. Edamame Beans

1 lb green bell peppers, sliced into wide strips

1 large red onion, cut into 1/2 inch thick rounds

1/3 cup Italian parsley or basil, finely chopped

Dressing Ingredients

6 tbsp. extra virgin olive oil

Sea salt, to taste

3 tbsp. Balsamic vinegar

1 tsp. Dijon mustard

Combine all of the dressing ingredients thoroughly.

Preheat your grill to low heat and grease the grates.

Layer the vegetables grill for 12 minutes per side, until tender flipping once.

Brush with the marinade/ dressing ingredients

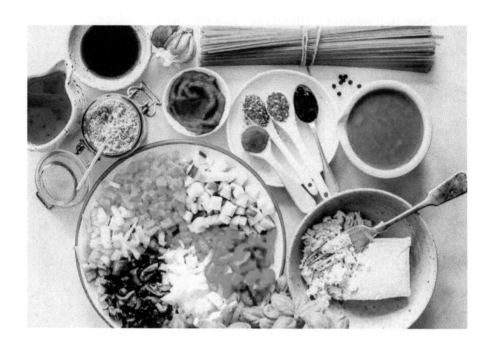

Grilled Baby Carrots and Green Bell Peppers

Ingredients

8 pcs. baby carrots

1 lb green bell peppers, sliced into wide strips

10 Broccolini Florets

10 pcs. Brussel Sprouts

1 large red onion, cut into 1/2 inch thick rounds

1/3 cup Italian parsley or basil, finely chopped

Dressing Ingredients

6 tbsp. extra virgin olive oil

Sea salt, to taste

1 tsp. onion powder

1/2 tsp. Herbs de Provence

3 tbsp. white vinegar

1 tsp. Dijon mustard

Combine all of the dressing ingredients thoroughly.

Preheat your grill to low heat and grease the grates.

Layer the vegetables grill for 12 minutes per side, until tender flipping once.

Brush with the marinade/ dressing ingredients

Grilled Artichoke Hearts and Baby Corn with honey vinaigrette

Ingredients

1 cup artichoke hearts

10 pcs. baby corn

1 bunch of Romaine Lettuce leaves

2 medium Carrots, cut lengthwise and cut in half

4 large Tomatoes, sliced thick

1/3 cup Italian parsley or basil, finely chopped

Dressing Ingredients

6 tbsp. extra virgin olive oil

Sea salt, to taste

3 tbsp. apple cider vinegar

1 tbsp. honey

1 tsp. Egg-free mayonnaise

Combine all of the dressing ingredients thoroughly.

Preheat your grill to low heat and grease the grates.

Layer the vegetables grill for 12 minutes per side, until tender flipping once.

Brush with the marinade/ dressing ingredients

Grilled Kale Beets and Carrots

Ingredients

1 bunch of Kale

5 pcs. Beets

2 medium Carrots, cut lengthwise and cut in half

4 large Tomatoes, sliced thick

1 large red onion, cut into 1/2 inch thick rounds

1/3 cup Italian parsley or basil, finely chopped

Dressing Ingredients:

6 tbsp. extra virgin olive oil

1 tsp. onion powder

Sea salt, to taste

3 tbsp. distilled white vinegar

1 tsp. Dijon mustard

Combine all of the dressing ingredients thoroughly.

Preheat your grill to low heat and grease the grates.

Layer the vegetables grill for 12 minutes per side, until tender flipping once.

Brush with the marinade/ dressing ingredients

Grilled Okra and Artichoke

Ingredients

10 pcs. Okra

1 pc. Artichoke

1 large red onion, cut into 1/2 inch thick rounds

1/3 cup Italian parsley or basil, finely chopped

Dressing Ingredients

6 tbsp. olive oil

3 dashes of Tabasco hot sauce

Sea salt, to taste

3 tbsp. white wine vinegar

1 tsp. Egg-free mayonnaise

Combine all of the dressing ingredients thoroughly.

Preheat your grill to low heat and grease the grates.

Layer the vegetables grill for 12 minutes per side, until tender flipping once.

Brush with the marinade/ dressing ingredients

Grilled Cabbage Okra and Red Onion

Ingredients

1 medium Cabbage sliced

10 pcs. Okra

1 large red onion, cut into 1/2 inch thick rounds

1/3 cup Italian parsley or basil, finely chopped

10 Broccolini Florets

10 pcs. Brussel Sprouts

Dressing Ingredients

6 tbsp. olive oil

1 tsp. garlic powder

1 tsp. onion powder

Sea salt, to taste

3 tbsp. white wine vinegar

1 tsp. English mustard

Combine all of the dressing ingredients thoroughly.

Preheat your grill to low heat and grease the grates.

Layer the vegetables grill for 12 minutes per side, until tender flipping once.

Brush with the marinade/ dressing ingredients

Grilled Edamame Beans and Cabbage

Ingredients

20 pcs. Edamame Beans

1 medium Cabbage sliced

1 bunch of Romaine Lettuce leaves

2 medium Carrots, cut lengthwise and cut in half

4 large Tomatoes, sliced thick

1/3 cup Italian parsley or basil, finely chopped

Dressing Ingredients

6 tbsp. olive oil

3 dashes of Tabasco hot sauce

Sea salt, to taste

3 tbsp. white wine vinegar

1 tsp. Egg-free mayonnaise

Combine all of the dressing ingredients thoroughly.

Preheat your grill to low heat and grease the grates.

Layer the vegetables grill for 12 minutes per side, until tender flipping once.

Brush with the marinade/ dressing ingredients

Grilled Artichoke , Carrots and Kale

Ingredients

1 pc. Artichoke

1 bunch of Kale

2 medium Carrots, cut lengthwise and cut in half

4 large Tomatoes, sliced thick

1large white onion, cut into 1/2-inch slices

Dressing Ingredients

6 tbsp. olive oil

3 dashes of Tabasco hot sauce

Sea salt, to taste

3 tbsp. white wine vinegar

1 tsp. Egg-free mayonnaise

Combine all of the dressing ingredients thoroughly.

Preheat your grill to low heat and grease the grates.

Layer the vegetables grill for 12 minutes per side, until tender flipping once.

Brush with the marinade/ dressing ingredients

Grilled Beets and Artichoke Hearts

Ingredients

5 pcs. Beets

1 cup artichoke hearts

1 bunch of Romaine Lettuce leaves

2 medium Carrots, cut lengthwise and cut in half

4 large Tomatoes, sliced thick

Dressing Ingredients

6 tbsp. olive oil

3 dashes of Tabasco hot sauce

Sea salt, to taste

3 tbsp. white wine vinegar

1 tsp. Egg-free mayonnaise

Combine all of the dressing ingredients thoroughly.

Preheat your grill to low heat and grease the grates.

Layer the vegetables grill for 12 minutes per side, until tender flipping once.

Brush with the marinade/ dressing ingredients

Grilled Asparagus with English Mustard Vinaigrette

INGREDIENTS

2 teaspoons finely grated lemon zest

2 tablespoon fresh lemon juice

1 tablespoon English mustard

¼ cup extra virgin olive oil, plus more

Sea salt, freshly ground pepper

2 large bunches thick asparagus, trimmed

2 bunches spring onions, halved if large

 Preheat grill for medium-high heat.

Combine lemon zest, lemon juice, mustard, and ¼ cup oil in a bowl

Season with salt and pepper.

Place the asparagus and spring onions on a pan and drizzle with oil.

Season with sea salt and pepper.

Grill for about 4 minutes per side or until tender.

Sprinkle the dressing over the grilled vegetables.

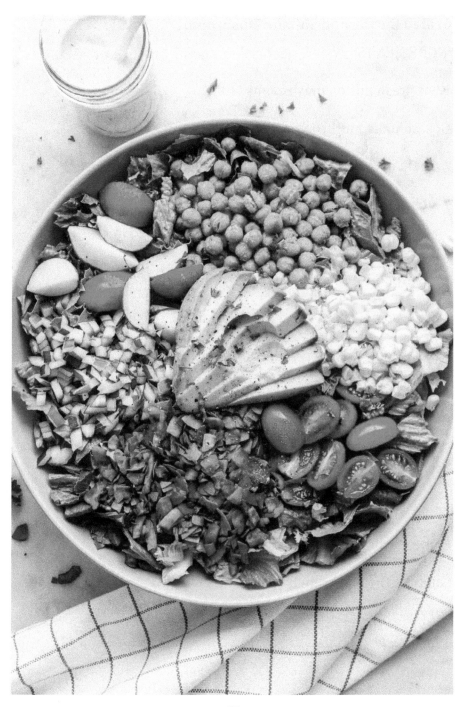

Grilled Button and Shitake Mushroom

INGREDIENTS

12 oz. fresh button mushrooms

4 oz. shiitake mushrooms

8 oz. small carrots (about 6), scrubbed, halved lengthwise.

4 tablespoons canola oil, divided

Sea salt and freshly ground black pepper

2 tablespoons reduced-sodium soy sauce

2 tablespoons unseasoned rice vinegar

1 tablespoon toasted sesame oil

1 teaspoon finely grated peeled ginger

6 scallions, thinly sliced on a diagonal

2 teaspoons toasted sesame seeds

Preheat grill for medium-high heat.

Combine the mushrooms and carrots with 3 Tbsp. canola oil in a bowl.

Season with salt and pepper.

Grill, while turning the mushrooms and carrots frequently, until tender.

Combine the soy sauce, vinegar, sesame oil, ginger, and remaining 1 Tbsp. canola oil in a bowl.

Cut the carrots into 2 inch long pieces

Cut the mushrooms into bite-size pieces.

Combine them with the vinaigrette, scallions and sesame seeds

Season with salt and pepper.

Grilled Cauliflower with Chipotle

INGREDIENTS

½ cup olive oil, plus more for grill

1 large head of cauliflower (about 2½ pounds), trim the stems and outer leaves removed.

2 canned chipotle chilies in adobo, finely chopped, plus 3 tablespoons adobo sauce

8 garlic cloves, finely grated

6 tablespoons red wine vinegar

3 tablespoons honey

2 tablespoons kosher salt

2 tablespoons smoked paprika

1 tablespoon dried oregano

Lemon wedges (for serving)

Prepare your grill for medium-low heat and oil the grates.

Slice the cauliflower into 4 equal parts.

Add the chilies, adobo sauce, garlic, vinegar, molasses, salt, paprika, oregano, and remaining ½ cup olive oil in a medium bowl to combine.

Brush this sauce on one side of each cauliflower steak and place steaks, sauce side down, on grill.

Brush the second side with sauce.

Grill the cauliflower until tender for 7–8 minutes.

Drizzle the cooked side with sauce

Grill until second side softens, 7–8 minutes.

Move to indirect heat, and brush with the sauce. C

Grill until tender. This takes about 20 minutes.

Serve with lemon wedges.

Grilled Asparagus with Miso

INGREDIENTS

¼ cup plus 2 tablespoons mirin (sweet Japanese rice wine)

¼ cup white miso

2 tablespoons seasoned white wine vinegar

2 teaspoons freshly grated peeled ginger

2 bunches asparagus (about 2 pounds), trimmed

lemon wedges, thinly sliced scallions, and toasted sesame seeds (for serving)

Sea salt , to taste

Prepare your grill for high heat.

Combine the mirin, miso, vinegar, and ginger in a bowl.

Layer the asparagus on a baking pan and pour the marinade mixture over.

Toss to combine.

Grill the asparagus until lightly charred and tender, 4 1/2 minutes.

Squeeze lime juice and garnish with scallions and sesame seeds.

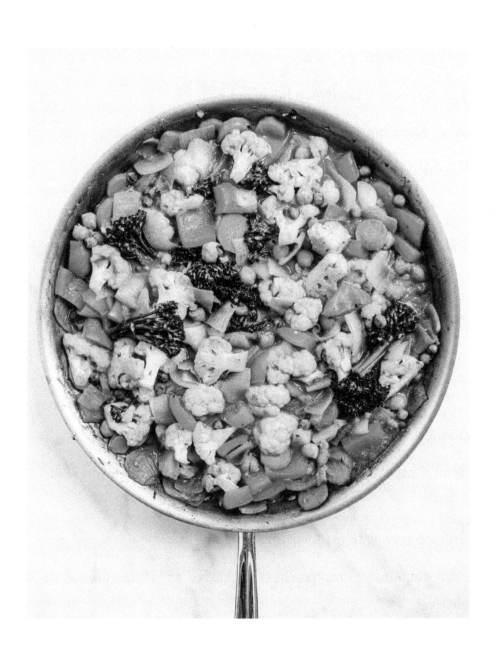

Grilled Corn with Poblano Chilies

INGREDIENTS

Olive oil (for grill)

2 tablespoons fresh lemon juice

¾ teaspoon hot sauce (such as Frank's)

Sea salt

4 ears of corn, in husk

2 small poblano chilies

3 tablespoons extra virgin olive oil

2 scallions, chopped

Preheat your grill for medium heat

Oil the grate.

Combine the lime juice and hot sauce in a bowl and season with salt.

Grill the corn with the husk on and chilies.

Turn frequently, until corn husk is charred and chilies are lightly charred

Drizzle corn with olive oil.

Cut the kernels.

Remove the seeds from chilies and chop finely.

Combine the corn with the scallions

Season with sea salt.

Grilled Broccoli with non-dairy yogurt

INGREDIENTS

2 small heads of broccoli (about 1½ pounds)

Sea salt

½ cup plain non-dairy yogurt

1 tablespoon olive oil

1 tablespoon English mustard

1½ teaspoons Kashmiri chili powder or paprika

1 teaspoon chaat masala

1 teaspoon ground cumin

1 teaspoon ground turmeric

Vegetable oil (for grill)

Trim the stems of the broccoli

Slice the stems lengthwise into ¼"-thick rectangles.

Break up the head of the broccoli into large florets.

Cook in a pot of boiling salted water until bright green and tender.
This takes 2 minutes.

Drain and transfer to a bowl of ice water.

Drain and pat dry.

Combine non-dairy yogurt, olive oil, mustard, chili powder, chaat masala, cumin, and turmeric in a large bowl.

Add the broccoli and combine with the liquid mixture.

Season with sea salt.

Prepare your grill for medium-high heat;.

Grill the broccoli until lightly charred in spots, 6 minutes.

Grilled Button Mushrooms with Almond Lemon Dip

INGREDIENTS

1½ cups whole blanched almonds

1 tablespoon fresh lemon juice

4 tablespoons extra virgin olive oil, divided

1 tablespoon plus 2 teaspoons sherry vinegar, divided

Sea salt

1 pound fresh button mushrooms, stems trimmed, halved lengthwise

Freshly ground black pepper

Preheat your oven to 350°.

Set 6 almonds aside for garnishing.

Toast the remaining nuts on a baking pan, toss frequently.

Roast until golden and aromatic. This takes about 8–10 minutes.

In a blender process the almonds until finely ground.

Add in lemon juice, 2 Tbsp. oil, 1 Tbsp. vinegar, and ½ cup water.

Blend by adding more water until dip becomes fairly smooth

Season with salt.

Prepare your grill for medium-high heat.

Combine mushrooms and remaining 2 Tbsp. oil in a bowl.

Season with salt and pepper.

Grill the mushrooms until tender and charred. This takes about 5 minutes.

Return the mushrooms to the bowl and combine with the remaining 2 tsp. vinegar.

Serve mushrooms with the dip and garnish with almonds.

Super Easy Grilled Fennel Bulbs

INGREDIENTS

4 medium fennel bulbs (about 3 pounds total), sliced lengthwise ½ inch thick

3 tablespoons extra virgin olive oil

Sea salt

Freshly ground pepper

Combine the fennel with the oil.

Season with sea salt and pepper.

Grill fennel over medium heat about 4 minutes each side.

Grilled Smoky Carrots with Vegan Yogurt

INGREDIENTS

3 pounds carrots with tops, scrubbed, tops trimmed to 1 inch

2 bunches scallions, tops trimmed, halved lengthwise

4 tablespoons extra virgin olive oil, divided

Sea salt

1 teaspoon cumin seeds

1 Serrano chili, finely chopped, plus more sliced for serving

1 cup plain non-dairy yogurt

3 tbsp. fresh lime juice

2 tablespoons chopped mint, plus leaves for serving

Special Equipment

A spice mill or mortar and pestle

Prepare your grill for medium-low heat.

Combine the carrots and spring onions on a rimmed baking pan with 2 Tbsp. olive oil

Season with sea salt.

Grill and cover, turning frequently tender, 15–20 minutes.

toast cumin in a pan over medium heat until fragrant.

Let it cool down.

Grind and mix this in a bowl together with chopped Serrano, yogurt, lime juice, chopped mint, and remaining 2 Tbsp. oil.

Season with sea salt.

Grilled Zucchini Mushroom and Cauliflower

INGREDIENTS Nutrition

2 zucchini, sliced

2 yellow squash, sliced

1 red pepper, cut into cubes

1 lb fresh button mushroom, halved

1 red onion, halved and sliced

2 cups broccoli florets

2 cups cauliflower florets

Vinaigrette Ingredients

lightly sprinkle with olive oil

3 tablespoons fresh lemon juice

9 garlic cloves

1 tablespoon chopped fresh basil

1/4 cup chopped parsley

¼ teaspoon oregano

Sea Salt

Pepper

Layer with vegetables on 2 pieces of aluminum foil.

Combine vinaigrette ingredients, drizzle over vegetables.

Cover and seal the aluminum foil

Grill while covered over medium heat for half an hour.

Turn the packets of aluminum foil once throughout the entire cooking process.

Grilled Cauliflower Broccoli and Asparagus

Ingredients

Cauliflower

Broccoli

Asparagus

½ cup extra virgin olive oil

1/2 tsp Italian seasoning

Sea Salt & pepper to taste

1/2 fresh lemon

Wash, drain and cut veggies.

For the Marinade combine:

Olive oil (1/8 cup)

Tuscan Herb olive oil (1/8 cup)

Italian seasoning (1/2 tsp.)

Sea salt & pepper to taste.

Marinate the cauliflower & broccoli florets with the marinade ingredients for 45 minutes in a zip top bag at room temperature.

Sprinkle the olive oil on the asparagus.

Season with 3/4 tsp. pepper and some sea salt to taste

Heat the grill to medium

Grill until vegetables become tender and crisp.

Squeeze the lemon juice over the vegetables

Grilled Carrots with Honey-Ginger Glaze

Ingredients

Vinaigrette Ingredients

1/4 cup honey

1/4 cup soy sauce

2 teaspoons freshly minced garlic, about 1 medium clove

1/2 teaspoon finely grated fresh ginger

1/4 teaspoon crushed red pepper flakes

For the Carrots:

3 large carrots, peeled and cut into 3/4-inch slices on a bias

3 tablespoons extra-virgin olive oil

1 scallion, thinly sliced

Sea salt

Combine the vinaigrette ingredients.

Combine the carrot slices with oil in a bowl.

Season with sea salt.

Preheat your grill and layer the carrots on the side of the grill to cook it gently with indirect heat for 45 min.

Make sure to flip the carrots every 15 min.

Brush with vinaigrette and grill.

Cook for 3 more minutes and move to a bowl.

Drizzle with vinaigrette and garnish with scallions

Grilled Spiraled Eggplants with Tomatoes

Ingredients

Filling Ingredients

1 1/2 cups non-dairy yogurt

1/2 cup finely vegan cheese

1 tablespoon fresh juice from 1 lemon

2 tsp. finely minced fresh oregano

1 teaspoon finely minced fresh mint

1 teaspoon finely minced fresh dill

1 teaspoon minced garlic (about 1 medium clove)

Sea salt and freshly ground black pepper

For the Eggplant Rolls:

2 large eggplants, ends trimmed and cut lengthwise into 1/4-inch slices

1/3 cup extra-virgin olive oil

3 Roma tomatoes, stemmed, cored, and cut into 1/4-inch dice

1 English cucumber, seeded and cut into 1/4-inch dice

Sea salt and freshly ground black pepper

Preheat your grill heat to medium-high

Combine the filling ingredients

Drizzle eggplants with olive oil, salt and pepper.

Grill eggplants on medium heat for 2 ½ min. each side.

Let it cool down for 4 min.

Spread the filling ingredients over each eggplant and top with tomatoes and cucumbers.

Roll the eggplants into spirals.

Grilled Zucchini Skewers

Vinaigrette Ingredients

1/4 cup extra virgin olive oil

2 tablespoons fresh lemon juice from 1 lemon, plus 1 additional lemon cut into wedges for serving

2 tablespoons white wine vinegar

4 teaspoons freshly minced garlic (about 2 medium cloves)

2 teaspoons dried oregano

1 teaspoon finely chopped fresh mint leaves

Sea salt and freshly ground black pepper

Main Ingredients

1 pound vegan cheese, cut into 3/4-inch cubes

2 medium zucchini, cut into into 1/2-inch rounds

2 medium red onions, peeled and cut into 3/4-inch chunks

1 pint grape tomatoes

Wooden skewers, soaked in water for at least 30 minutes prior to use

Tzatziki, for serving (optional)

Pita, warmed, for serving (optional)

Combine the vinaigrette Ingredients.

Skewer the cheese, zucchini, onion, and tomatoes.

Preheat your grill to medium.

Grill until the cheese melts and zucchini for 4 minutes or until it becomes tender.

Squeeze lemon juice and serve with the vinaigrette, tzatziki and pita bread.

Shishito Peppers Skewers With Teriyaki Glaze Recipe

Ingredients

1 pound shishito peppers

Sea salt

Freshly ground black pepper

1/4 cup teriyaki sauce

Skewer the peppers onto sets of 2 skewers, keeping each of them about 1 inch apart to make them easier to flip.

Preheat your grill to medium-high.

Grill each pepper until charred on one side, about 2 minutes.

Flip peppers and grill on the other side, about 2 minutes longer.

Season with salt and pepper.

Brush with teriyaki sauce.

Grilled Radicchio With Vegan Cheese

Ingredients

2 whole heads radicchio, split in half through core

Sea salt and freshly ground black pepper

1/3 cup crumbled vegan tofu-based cheese

Extra-virgin olive oil, for drizzling

Saba or balsamic syrup, for drizzling (see note)

Preheat your grill to medium high

Place radicchio cut side-down on the grill.

Grill until lightly charred on one side, about 2 minutes.

Flip and season the top with salt and pepper.

Grill the other side until it is charred, about 2 minutes longer.

Cook over indirect heat until fully tender, about 1 minute longer.

Sprinkle with vegan cheese

Drizzle with olive oil and syrup.

Avocado Beans and Tomato Bowl

Ingredients

1/2 cup Savory Stewed Black Beans, warmed

1 teaspoon extra-virgin olive oil

1/2 cup Roma tomatoes

1/4 cup fresh corn kernels (from 1 ear)

1/2 medium-sized ripe avocado, thinly sliced

1 medium radish, very thinly sliced

2 tablespoons fresh cilantro leaves

1/4 teaspoon sea salt

1/8 teaspoon black pepper

Heat the skillet over medium high heat.

Add oil to the pan.

Add tomatoes to the oil and cook until tender but charred for about 3 minutes.

Set the tomatoes beside the beans in a large bowl.

Cook the corn and cook for 2 ½ min.

Place the corn next to the tomatoes.

Add avocado, radish, and cilantro.

Season with salt and pepper.

Quinoa Black Bean Bowls

Ingredients

2 teaspoons extra-virgin olive oil, divided

1 teaspoon white wine vinegar

 1/4 teaspoon sea salt, divided

1 cup hot cooked quinoa

1 cup grape tomatoes, halved

1/2 cup canned unsalted black beans, rinsed, drained, and warmed

2 tablespoons chopped cilantro, plus more for garnish

1/2 ripe avocado, sliced

Combine 1 1/2 teaspoons oil, vinegar, and dash of sea salt.

Mix the quinoa, tomatoes, beans, cilantro, and 1/8 teaspoon salt thoroughly.

Divide this mixture between 2 bowls.

Heat a pan over medium heat.

Add the remaining 1/2 teaspoon oil.

Crack eggs, 1 at a time, into your pan.

Cover and let it cook until the whites are set and yolk is still runny, takes about 2 to 3 minutes.

Pour the dressing evenly over quinoa mixture

Garnish with eggs and avocado.

Season with remaining dash of sea salt.

Garnish with cilantro.

Brussels Sprouts with Soy Dressing

Ingredients

2 tablespoons sesame oil, divided

4 ounces tempeh, thinly sliced

4 teaspoons l soy sauce

2 teaspoons sherry vinegar

1/8 teaspoon sea salt

2 tablespoons chopped fresh cilantro, divided

11/2 cups very thinly sliced Brussels sprouts

Thin jalapeno chili slices

2 tablespoons chopped unsalted peanuts, toasted

2 lime wedges

Heat a pan over medium-high

Heat 1 tablespoon of the oil in the pan.

Add tempeh and cook until very crisp and browned, takes about 2 minutes per side.

Transfer to a plate.

Combine the soy sauce, vinegar, salt, 1 tablespoon of the cilantro, and the remaining sesame oil in a bowl.

Add the Brussels sprouts, and mix to coat.

Divide between 2 bowls.

Sprinkle with jalapeno chili slices and peanuts, and top with the tempeh slices.

Pour the remaining dressing, and top with the remaining cilantro.

Serve with lime wedges.

Vegan Teriyaki Noodles

Ingredients

¼ cup soy sauce

1 tablespoon honey (coconut nectar, or coconut/brown sugar, add more or less to taste)

1 teaspoon rice vinegar

½ teaspoon sesame oil

pinch of black pepper (can use crushed red pepper or sriracha if you like it more spicy)

8–9 oz ramen noodles

2 cups shredded Napa cabbage or other green leafy vegetable like baby bok choy, spinach, or regular cabbage

3 carrots, julienned

1 whole green bell pepper, stem and seeds discarded and thinly sliced (any color will do)

4-5 mushrooms, sliced (baby bella, shiitake, button, etc.)

3 cloves garlic, minced

1 cup snow peas

3–4 green onions, chopped into 2-inch pieces

Place noodles into a pot of boiling water and cook just until the noodles start to break up.

Take it off the heat, drain and rinse with cold water.

To Make Sauce:

Combine the soy sauce, honey, rice vinegar, sesame oil, and pepper.

Heat the oil over medium-high heat.

Add the cabbage, carrots, bell pepper, mushrooms, and garlic.

Sauté vegetables for 2 1/2 minutes until tender.

Add snow peas and green onions and sauté for another minute.

Add the noodles and half of the sauce.

Stir-fry on high heat for 1 ½ minutes until sauce thickens and coats the noodles.

Add the remaining sauce.

Vegan Spaghetti Carbonara

Ingredients

Cashew Sauce:

1 cup of cashews (soaked overnight)

3/4 cup vegetable broth

2 tbsp nutritional yeast

3 cloves of garlic minced

1 red onion minced

Sea salt

Pepper

Carbonara:

250 g whole-wheat spaghetti pasta

300 g white close cup mushrooms (sliced)

1 cup green peas (fresh or frozen)

1 small red onion (minced)

3 clove garlic (minced)

1- 2 tbsp extra-virgin olive oil

fresh parsley

Sea salt

Black pepper

To Make The Cashew Cheese

Wash the cashews and process in a blender with the rest of ingredients.

Blend until you have smooth texture.

To Make The Spaghetti Carbonara

Cook your pasta according to the package instructions.

Drizzle with olive oil.

Heat olive oil in a pan with medium heat.

Add garlic and stir fry for 1 minute.

Add onion and mushrooms and stir fry until brown (for about 5 mins.).

Add peas and cook further for 3 mins.

Stir in ¼ cup of cashew cheese

Garnish with fresh parsley.

Rice Noodle Salad

Ingredients

Sauce

3 tbsp Soy Sauce

1 tbsp Rice Wine Vinegar

1 tbsp Honey

1 tsp Lemon Juice

Salad

100 g Rice Noodles

1 Carrot

1 Zucchini

1/4 Purple Cabbage finely sliced

1 Green Bell Pepper finely sliced

1 Yellow Pepper finely sliced

1 bunch Fresh Coriander roughly chopped

1 small handful Cashew Nuts roughly chopped

1 tsp Sesame Seeds

1/2 Red Chili

Combine all of the sauce ingredients.

Soak the noodles according to the instructions in the packaging.

Combine with the carrots and zucchini.

Add all of the remaining finely chopped veggies in.

Combine with the sauce, and garnish with the coriander, cashews, sesame seeds and chili.

.

Vegan Spaghetti Bolognese

Ingredients

200 grams (7 oz) spaghetti

1 medium zucchini , spiralized

1 medium red onion, diced

6 cloves of garlic, minced

2 cups (480 ml) tomato sauce

2 cups (340 grams) cooked lentils

1 ½ teaspoons Spanish paprika

2 teaspoons oregano

2 teaspoon red wine vinegar

½ teaspoon sea salt

A few grinds of pepper

Cook the pasta according to the package instructions.

Heat a pan over medium-high heat.

Add the onion, garlic, and some water.

Stir fry until soft and add the rest of the ingredients

Cook until the lentils are heated.

Toss the pasta together with the zucchini.

Pour the lentil Bolognese sauce.

Tomatoes Stuffed With Pesto

Ingredients

Pesto Cream

2 large bunches basil (about 2 cups lightly packed leaves)

1/4 cup extra virgin olive oil

1/4 cup raw cashews, soaked

1 garlic clove

1 tsp nutritional yeast

Sea salt and pepper to taste

Quinoa Filling

1 tbsp extra virgin olive oil

1 medium red onion, diced

10 oz fresh spinach

3 garlic cloves

1/2 tsp Italian seasoning

3 cups cooked quinoa

6 Tbsp vegan pesto

Sea salt

Black pepper to taste

Tomatoes -

6 large tomatoes, (seeds and cores scooped out)

2 Tbsp extra virgin olive oil

Sea salt and pepper to taste

fresh basil

Preheat your oven to 400 degrees F.

Combine all of the pesto ingredients in a blender and blend until smooth.

In a pan, sauté the onion in olive oil for 7 minutes or until translucent.

Add the spinach and garlic cloves and cook for 2 more minutes .

Add the cooked quinoa, pesto sauce, Italian seasonings, salt, and pepper.

Cut the top of each tomatoes. Scoop out all the seeds.

Drizzle olive oil in a baking pan and spread it around.

Place the tomatoes in the baking pan and drizzle with a tbsp of oil over the top of the tomatoes.

Season with salt & pepper.

Ladle the pesto quinoa filling into each of the tomatoes and put the tops back on.

Roast for 30 minutes.

Garnish with basil.